Sugar Detox for Beginners

Lose Weight, Gain Energy, and Level Mood Naturally

By Rebecca Lewis

© 2015

Table of Contents

Introduction

SHOCKER! The U.S. Department of Agriculture reports the average American eats over 156 pounds of added sugar. And because sugar has become so abundant in the foods we eat it's next to impossible to recognize how consumed we are in it.

If you translate this into daily consumption, the Centers for Disease Control reports the average American gets almost 30 teaspoons per day, equating to about 440 calories. This is almost 25% of the typical 2000 calorie diet intake. On occasion that wouldn't be the end of the world. Unfortunately because of the proven addictive nature of sugar it's incredibly difficult to say no after your first bite. And the more you eat the more impossible it is to to stop. Some people call it a poison because that's exactly what added sugar does to your health over time.

FACT - Research shows refined added sugars like you'll find in processed fast foods, cakes, muffins, cookies, white breads and soda, negatively affect the chemical balance within your body and how your brain works. And both physical and mental processes are strong influencers of your sugar addiction.

The great news is that by taking a step by step approach and committing to remove sugar from your life completely, you can succeed and reap the rewards. Some of which are long-term energy gain, decreased risk of serious disease, improved thinking, level blood sugars and mood, increased positivity, weight loss, and a strengthened immune system.

And important to note is you are going to have to understand how to create new positive habits so you can slowly but surely replace your unhealthy sugar fixes.

Effective Pointers to Create New Healthy Habits

*Set reasonable expectations - Understand nobody is perfect and one food at a time is perfectly fine if that's what works for you.

*Understand why you are giving up sugar - If you can focus on the logical when your sugar cravings smack you it's much easier to talk yourself out of giving in.

*Look for other connections - People use sugar for all sorts of reasons other than nutrition. Which of course isn't the case because added sugar isn't nutrition. Search for the reasons you eat sugar and why so you can use this information to help you eliminate sugar.

*Write down your new goals - Seeing is believing and great for reminding you of your intentions when you slip off course.

*Make sure you get support - Talk about quitting sugar with your friends and family, doctor and fitness trainer. Knowing you have a support circle in place will inspire you to make it happen.

*Set a reasonable timeline - You know yourself best. If you know taking the long route to zapping sugar is best for you then make sure you set up your plan of action with this consideration. If you know that it's all or nothing with you then that's what you need to do. Be smart and use tactics that will work for you.

*Be prepared to fall - Nobody is perfect and it's really tough to make changes. As humans we are creatures of habit good and bad. We find comfort in things we know are harmful simply because they are comfortable and we are used to them. Commit to making sure you are going to kick the sugar habit and be forgiving of yourself when on occasion you indulge. Let it go. Get back on track and move forward with a smile.

This introductory sugar addiction guide gives you the knowledge and take-action information you need to forget sugar and start living your life sugar-free and fantastic!

And keep in mind even if you eliminate even half of the added sugars in your diet you're a winner because that's ten steps closer to better optimal health, where every step matters. You control YOU, nobody else. Decide to kick the sugar habit and I'll help you get started!

Chapter 1 - Types of Sugar and Sugar Addiction

HealthlineNews experts report sugar is a drug that is just as powerful as a medical prescription, street drug, or alcohol.

It's critical that you understand the different types of sugar before we get into how sugar addiction negatively affects your life; physically, mentally, socially, and emotionally. A powerful food that will sneak up and silently take control of your moods, thoughts, actions, and how your physical appearance.

There are many different types of sugars. Some used for specialty baking and not available in the grocery store. The size of the crystals and textures vary giving each a unique properties, look, and purpose. In a nutshell the main types of sugar are white, brown, and liquid, according to The Sugar Association.

WHITE SUGAR

This is the most common sugar type. Otherwise known as table sugar or granulated sugar. I'm sure you've used it in baking cookies, sprinkled on strawberries, or when making fruity punch. It's ground extra fine so there won't be any clumping and it mixes easily.

Bakers Sugar - This sugar is especially fine for specialty baking projects. It's often for the sugar topping on cakes and donuts.

Fruit Sugar - It's a touch finer than granulated sugar and used in numerous dry mixes, desserts, and puddings.

Bar Sugar - This is the finest type of sugar used for things like meringue and sweet drinks because it's light and dissolves readily.

Powdered Sugar - This sugar is white sugar grounded down and then sifted. It's often used to sprinkle on to of French toast or pancakes, and icings and whipping cream.

Sanding Sugar - This sparkly sugar has larger crystals and is used on top of cookies, cakes and pastries.

Coarse Sugar - Is a larger crystal sugar that holds its structure when cooking and baking. You'll find it in syrups for liquors or fondants.

BROWN SUGAR

These sugars have some processing and range from light to ultra-dark in color. Some people sprinkle brown sugar on their oatmeal or bake with it.

Turbinado Sugar - The washing process of this brown sugar takes some of the molasses off and lightens it. The flavor is mild and you may have used this in your tea or other drinks.

Brown Sugar (dark/light) - This is a common sugar that keeps some of the molasses which gives the deep pleasurable flavor and unique "wettish" texture. The darker the color the stronger the molasses flavor. Baked beans, gingerbread, and baking often uses brown sugar. Keep in mind if you leave the bag open this sugar will harden because it's got lots of moisture.

Cane Juice (evaporated) - This is a free-flowing light colored sugar with a touch of molasses flavor. This juice is clarified first and then evaporated into syrup. Then it's crystalized and cured.

Barbados Sugar - A dark brown sugar with a strong molasses flavor. It's stickier than normal brown sugar.

Brown Sugars (free flowing) - A co-crystallization processed is used to make less moist powdery brown sugar. It's great for baking.

Demerara Sugar - A hit in England, this sugar has slightly sticky large molecules. It's popular on cereals and for tea time.

LIQUID SUGAR - These are dissolved sugars that are often used when the sugar needs to be in liquid form. It's a dark color and is used where a dark appearance is required.

Invert Sugar - Glucose and fructose make up sucrose. This conversion process to create sucrose is often used in commercial baking where it's ideal to have equal parts of glucose and fructose. Invert sugar tastes sweeter than table sugar because it has fructose, which is sweeter than granulated sugar.

At home if a recipe calls for boiling sugar in lemon water, invert sugar is created.

That's it for the basic types of sugars. Now we're going to move into what sugar addiction is.

Sugar Addiction

You don't need the food science experts at BBC Science to tell you sugar is chemically addictive. We are taught from childhood that sugary sweets are a devilishly good treat. We are taught to crave them because they are treated like the forbidden fruit. And everyone wants what they can't have right?

You go from sneaking cookies to taking a bite of that bittersweet baking chocolate in your mom's cupboard. We get all excited for desert and extra sweet treats around the holidays.

In general we are taught to crave sugar and when your taste buds get ahold of it you just want more and more and more.

Sugar Addiction is...

Technically the state of addiction to eating sugar.

Scientists believe our body naturally craves sugar because intrinsically you need it for survival. But it is natural sugars from fresh fruit and natural sweeteners like honey (for non-vegans) that we need. Not the sugar loaded diets of processed foods, cakes, muffins, pastries, fast foods, and candy that we pig out on.

Expert researchers have found out taste buds search out salt, fat, and sugar. The problem is we don't seem to understand natural and moderation and this gets us into hot water.

Unless your body is forced into a state of ketosis it uses the glucose readily available in your bloodstream and converts it into energy to be absorbed by your cells. Glucose is critical for brain function because it's the main energy source. Your nerve cells need a constant supply of glucose in order to function optimally. Unfortunately your body can't store glucose for long periods of time so you need a constant supply or you can quickly hit the danger zone of low blood glucose levels. That can lead to coma and death in extreme cases.

Did you know...?

Researchers from Washington University conducted a study on newborns indicating sweets were preferred.

Serious Issue - Sugary foods are far too readily available. Temptation is constant 24/7. One reason why obesity rates in children continue to climb. The Childhood Obesity Foundation states in 2013 over 42 million infants and children were overweight or obese and by 2025 experts believe without intervention that number will climb to 70 million.

Main Reason People Binge on Sugar

It temporarily and instantaneously lifts your spirits. Sugar triggers a serotonin release that puts a smile on your face. From here we create an emotional connection that has zippo to do with being hungry.

The flip side is your dose of sugar also signals to your brain to release insulin to try and level your blood sugar spike. This is hard on your liver and kidneys and kicks you into a crash. This fuels the desire to want more sugar to enter Happy-Ville again.

A cycle of sugar addiction destruction has been created -

Naturally your body has a tough time gauging when you've had enough processed simple sugars because technically they are a foreign substance and not programmed into your body.

The technical of it according to experts at Yale University is that glucose actually temporarily suppresses parts of the brain wanting you to eat but fructose doesn't. Fructose increases the chances of you overeating and glucose leaves you more satisfied.

Many foods have hidden sugars and most processed food have at least half of the sugar as addictive fructose. And because your body can't scientifically decipher between processed sugar, honey, fruit sugar or dairy sugar, it makes it very difficult to control your sugar intake.

*No more than 10% of calories should come from sugar each day. For men this is about 15 teaspoons and women 13 teaspoons. That's like having 2 cans of soda or 8 cookies.

Sugar addiction is a serious issue that affects millions of people world-wide. Increasing the risk of obesity, heart disease, stroke, diabetes, and all sorts of other deadly illnesses. Let's have a look at how to kick the sugar habit when you're ready!

Chapter 2 - How to Bust Sugar Cravings - Better Food Choices

Step One - Having courage to recognize you have a sugar addiction and WANTING to take action.

Step Two - Gain the knowledge required to create your plan and make it happen.

Psychology Today experts say it takes more than 6 months of repeating an action to make it habit. That's where you don't have to focus so intensely on the new action. Change is tough and we are resistant to it.

FACT - If you want to leave your sugar cravings at the candy store you are going to have to crave change and make it stick. You are In control of you so ultimately there's nobody to point the finger at but yourself if you decide to jump ship and not climb back on.

There are lots of different tactics and strategies to get sugar off your plate and out of your mind. Here are a few to get you started.

Give Yourself a Taste - WebMD dietitians believe you should start by giving yourself a little. Most people fail because they try to go cold turkey, shock their system, and quickly slip back into their unhealthy habits. Have a two bites of cake or a mini chocolate bar. If you are feeling completely deprived you are more likely to fail.

Try Finding Combinations - This one is just like sitting on the fence. You are looking to get the nutritious with a little treat. Have a few strawberries dipped in chocolate. Or a sprinkle of brown sugar on your oatmeal. A nut mixture with a few smarties in it really hits the spot. This will help you crave healthy foods and the extras will soon fade away.

Flip the Switch - This is a tough move. Just be wary the first few days afterwards you may be feeling a little "off." Depending on how much sugar your body was used to. Your cravings will dissipate but you have to be willing to wait it out.

Turn Up the Fruit Volume - Initially this may seem like a cheap consolation prize. Out of your Halloween treat bag do you want an apple or a peanut butter cup? By eating more fruit you will curb your craving for fructose faster. And if you stick with it long enough you're going to start craving all-natural ripe and tasty fruit!

Stock Up On Sugar-Free Gum - Health professionals across the board are going to back this one. For some people it's boredom that triggers sugar cravings. Chewing on gum keeps your mouth and mind busy.

Take Up a New Hobby - I call this one the distraction method. If you start thinking about chocolate ice-cream or fresh baked cookies go hop on your horse or practice your golf swing. Get excited about something new in your life to help forget about sugar.

Get Support - It's funny in life how many times we are okay with disappointing ourselves but we're not so good with letting other people down. Shout it out to the world your commitment to knock excess sugar out of your life and let your cheerleaders help keep you on track.

Eat every 3-4 Hours - By making sure you eat small meals regularly you'll keep your blood sugars level and ward off sugar cravings. Willpower gets incredibly difficult on an empty stomach.

Get Back On Your Horse - If you happen to fall when you're out with friends and decide to eat a big ice-cream sundae, or you dive into the cookie one night when you were feeling bummed, pick yourself up and move on. Don't worry about it because we all steer off course from time to time. One slip up won't kill you. Just make sure it's the exception to the rules.

I personally am **vegan** and I know it's not easy for everyone to adapt to the vegan lifestyle. I only eat natural plant based foods. So I am going to make things easier for you by giving you healthier options. Hopefully with time you'll gradually make a transition into veganism should you choose a healthier lifestyle.

Now we are going to have a look at sugary food options that are better. It's all about making smaller healthier choices step by step.

Unhealthy	Healthier
Packaged cinnamon Danish	Whole grain toast with sugar cinnamon
Strawberry Pop Tart	1/2 whole wheat bagel with jam
Sugar cereal	Steel cut oats with fresh berries
Carmel corn	Nuts
Chips	Air popped popcorn
Candy bar	All-natural granola bar
Corn chips	Rice cakes
Smarties	Raisins
Chocolate sauce	Honey
Ice-cream	Sugar-free frozen yogurt
Soda	Diet soda
Chocolate chip muffin	Muesli cookie
Cookie	All-natural oat bar
Nutella on crackers	Celery sticks with peanut butter
Jell-O	Sugar-free gelatin
Candy	Pineapple
Juice	Sugar-free carbonated water
Chocolate pie	Yogurt and fresh berries
Chocolate almond	Nut mixture with dried fruit
Chocolate pudding	Fresh fruit
Donut	Whole grain English muffin - Jam
Caramel apple	Apples dipped in peanut butter

Use these food examples as a platform from which to get started. You aren't trying to be perfect. Just aim to make better food decisions today than you did yesterday. Having the take-action knowledge to zap sugar is your first step. Life is a journey and the foods you eat each day reflect on how you think, feel, act, and view yourself, people around you, and your life in general. Use these pointers to help open your mind to change and when you are ready start applying.

Chapter 3 - Sugar Detox Basics

If you are going to successfully remove sugar from the cells and tissue within your body you're going to have to purge your

system of it and slowly fill it back up with wholesome macronutrients, and vitamins and minerals to build your body and

 mind strong, while providing optimal energy and resistance to disease.

You will need to stop eating excess sugar and detox of cleanse your body of it.

First, here are a few negative consequences of sugars according to nutritionists at Chatelaine.com...

*Interfere with immune system function

*Increase blood fats (triglycerides)

*Increase depression, anxiety, hyperactivity, and memory issues

*Raises "bad" (LDL) cholesterol and raising "good" (HDL) cholesterol

*Increases risk of high blood pressure and cholesterol

*Supports tooth decay and dental hygiene issues

*Triggers diabetes

*Increases the natural aging process and encourages wrinkles

*Causes obesity

*May trigger toxemia in pregnancy

*Boosts risk of fatty liver disease

*Causes bloating and tummy troubles

*Triggers headaches, migraines, and TMJ pain

*Causes bowel issues

*Boosts risk of specific cancers and disease

*Contributes to Alzheimer's

Here are a few steps to help you kick your sugar addiction:

Step One - Recognition

Professor of Medicine and Nutritional Science at the University of Wisconsin, Richard Atkinson, reports scientific studies prove sugar is more than 8 times as addictive a cocaine. Sugar has the power to alter your brain chemistry. The way you think, act, feel, and perceive.

It's really quite simple to test this theory out for yourself. If you are used to having an afternoon snack of a pop and chocolate bar, try going without. If your body is used to this habit of sugar induction you will feel de-energized and down if you miss it. Or you can just monitor your mood before and after you eat something sugary. The body can't help but shoot up with energy temporarily because of the short-lived energy from the simple sugars you've just ingested. Which also plummets just as quickly as it boosted your mood.

Step Two - Understanding

If you make the time to understand how and why your body reacts so strongly to sugar this will help you take action against it. The science of it all can get very confusing. In a nutshell your gut contains over 100 million neurons and numerous neurotransmitters just like your brain.

Almost all of your serotonin is in your bowels. Serotonin helps you feel good or relief. Think of it as comfort or safety. Food is created to comfort you. Some people are predisposed with low serotonin levels, which makes the quick comfort from refined sugars much more magnetic.

Endorphins are also released to relieve pain and if you eat sugar you're releasing beta-endorphin, which makes you want more sugar. So the more sugary food you eat the more you will want. A never ending cycle of destruction. And when you eat the physical act releases dopamine which also helps comfort you.

What happens is over time you need to eat more refined sugar in order to achieve the same levels of dopamine. Creating a "more and more" cycle.

Fact - the only way to break this progressive destructive cycle is to quit!

Step Three - Degree of Addiction

There are tests online or you can go through your doctor to find out exactly what degree of sugar addiction you have. This will dictate whether or not you are a candidate for stopping cold turkey or whether or not you may need to do it in stages.

Step Four - Know Sugar Foods

So many foods have hidden sugars. You are going to have to become a master of reading food labels so you know exactly what foods have sugars and which ones don't. Your best option is to cancel out all processed foods but often this isn't practical. At least not initially. It's important you set yourself up for success by learning which foods are best for you and how to make better substitutions until you reach your final goal of zero sugar in your diet.

Step Five - Study What You Can and Can't Eat

If you don't take the time to find which foods have sugar that you eat and which ones don't, it's impossible for you to kick the sugar habit. One great route I suggest is to journal everything you eat for the week. Then you can sit down and figure out systematically where your sugar is coming from. When you have this information you are ready to start zapping sugar from your plate.

Step Six - Purge Your Cupboards, Fridge, and House of Sugar

If you have sugary foods within reach you are much more likely to eat them. If you have sugar in the house just the smell or sight of it can trigger your craving. If you can't see it that's going to help you UN-learn wanting it. This also gives you a few minutes to think hard about your craving when it strikes. Do you really want to get dressed, hop in the car, and head down to the variety store to buy a candy bar? NO YOU DON'T!

Step Seven - Cut Out Sugar

Behavioral research shows the most successful route to kick sugar addiction is to remove it altogether. Some people are okay with moderation by many others aren't. If you are like me you've got an "all or nothing" mentality. Give me the whole piece of cake or none at all.

Try detoxing first on either a 10 or 30 day sugar detox program and then see how you feel. The majority of people that do this feel like they have control of their sugar and the cravings have diminished.

The most important factor here is that you find a lifestyle plan that works for you and either eliminates or reduces sugar. You've got to find your plan for life.

Step Eight - Plan Your Eating

If you plan what you are going to eat before you're hungry, the odds of success are much higher. When we are starving our willpower seems to shoot down the drain. Variety is the spice of life and by taking control of what you eat and putting the time in to create your meals, you're going to enjoy them so much more. This also gives you the control to create meals void of sugar, which is exactly what the doctor ordered!

Step Nine - Recognize Temptation and Build a Defense

You know your weaknesses, preferences and tolerances. It's up to you to remove sugar temptation from your life. Particularly the first month you are kicking sugar out the back door. You may have to skip the girls Friday night shopping if you know the tradition is to indulge in ice-cream and chocolate. Maybe your ultimate weakness is walking by the bakery every morning on route to work. So you'll just have to take another route that goes miles away from your weak spot.

Work with the facts and don't dangle the sugar carrot in front of yourself. That just makes sense.

Step Ten - Plan a Cleanse

If you are addicted to sugar your blood, tissues, and organs are loaded with it and extra toxic substances your body doesn't know how to get rid of. By committing to at least a 10-day sugar detox plan you will give yourself a head start trying to get rid of these built up sugars in your system. By removing them totally you will help starve the craving.

After you have flushed all the sugar out of your body you can fill it up with essential vitamins and minerals, protein, good carbs, and good fat to help build your body strong, level blood sugars, keep your moods level and deter serious disease like diabetes from setting in.

Step Eleven - Maintain

Making change is difficult. Have a plan in place to remind you of your goals and support you in achieving them. A diary works great to see your progress and this also gives you the visual and when and how you got side-tracked.

Having friends and family reminding you of what your goals are is always great. And for many people I suggest having a professional that you check in with regularly like a nutritionist, fitness expert, or even your doctor. This will help you hold accountability for your hard work and sugar detox goals.

Having a plan in place to remove sugar from your world is VIP important. Everyone is different and whether you take small baby steps or a gigantic leap through the process, as long as you are moving forward you are winning. Make the time to create your plan and commit to seeing it through. You deserve to be healthy and happy and sugar isn't invited.

Chapter 4 - Weight Loss and Sugar Connection

Mercola.com experts report most people that remove or drastically reduce sugar from their diet are going to lose weight. This is inevitable because when you are removing fatty processed and high sugar foods from your diet this means you are taking in fewer calories. When you eat fewer calories you're going to lose weight. The numbers don't lie.

Balancing your blood sugar levels is essential for overall fitness and well-being, healthy hormones, directing your body to burn more stored fat, and boosting your metabolism to shed pounds, according to Dr. Oz. What happens is people make a habit of eating unhealthy sugary processed foods that trigger repeated spikes in blood sugars. This not only affects your mood and increased risk of disease, but it also interferes in your ability to lose weight. With high blood sugar levels you are communicating to your body to store more fat and not burn it. On the flip side if you are not getting enough calories your body slips into starvation mode where it hoards all calories instead of burning them. A balance is important and that comes from removing extra sugars and eating a healthy well-balanced diet.

Pointers to Level Blood Sugar

1 - Get rid of extra unnatural sugars. Your body doesn't need it and these refined sugars just stress your system. The only way you can remove the high glucose spikes is to get rid of the sugar.

2 - Eating regularly, every 3-4 hours, will give your body a constant supply of energy that is level and doesn't push your energy levels too high or too low.

3 - What you eat is incredibly important. Filling your plate full of fresh vegetables is priority one. Add to this small portions of lean protein like wild salmon, eggs, and nuts. And small amounts of legumes and whole grains. Healthy fats like avocado, olive oil and coconut oil are also essential to fat burn and optimal brain function.

Choosing whole organic foods in the proper amount while balancing your plate is the best move you can make to kick sugar, blast fat, and get energized.

4 - Have healthy snacks with you at all times. Keep them in your purse, car, briefcase, and at the office just in case!

*Cheese string

*Beef jerky

*Greek yogurt with small handful sunflower seeds

*All-natural protein bar

*Apples, pears, and bananas

*Mixed almonds and raisins (1/2 cup)

*Sliced veggies (carrots, celery, cucumber, and peppers)

*Organic granola bar

*Peanut butter and Romaine lettuce on whole wheat tortilla (no mess!)

*Dried fruit (1/2 cup)

*Bottled water

5 - Exercising daily is important for level blood sugars. It's essential to work your slow twitch and fast twitch muscles if you want to burn fat all over. You can do this by making sure you get explosive high intensity exercise along with steady cardiovascular training daily. An example would be exploding up a flight of stairs and then biking around the block a few times.

You should aim for 30 minutes of cardiovascular activity each day with weight training/strength training 3 days a week for about 20 minutes. This helps build lean muscle to blast fat and keep your heart and lungs strong, while toning and strengthening your body.

According to nutrition experts at Oprah.com there are very few people, aside from diabetics, that have serious issues with their blood sugars. In order for your body cells to function nicely they want plenty of readily available, easily sucked up glucose floating in your blood and cells. This keeps your brain fueled and heart thumping.

Simultaneously while all your muscle and organs are singing in perfect harmony. Your hormone system is supposed to keep blood sugars level but you will mess this up eating too many simple carbohydrate sugary foods, like candy, soda, white bread, pasta and rice, cakes, cookies and pastries, and other processed high-fat food choices.

Slow and steady wins the race here. You need to teach your body to crave healthy complex carbs including whole grain pasta, rice and bread, veggies, beans, and legumes. Long lasting muscle building lean protein like eggs, fish, meat, poultry, quinoa, beans and nuts, are excellent for leveling the sugar in your blood and triggering weight loss.

You should also incorporate healthy fats in moderation to help satiate hunger and leave you fuller longer. Adding avocado to your salad or stir-fry is great, drizzling olive oil or cooking with grapes seed oil or coconut oil is excellent. Stay away from vegetable oils for cooking because they start oxidizing at low temperatures. Which means you are putting unhealthy substances into your body.

By knocking sugar out of your diet you will open up the door to losing weight fast and heading towards great health for life!

P.S. – Don't forget about serving sizes when you are looking to lose weight. If you think restaurant portions are what your body needs you better give your head a rattle! Healthy Living nutritionist's state restaurants typically serve 2-3 times more food than your body needs! A smart move is to ask for a doggy bag before your meal comes and immediately put half of it away

to take home or give to someone that would appreciate it. Makes for an easy dinner!

For non-vegans here are some typical portions:

Typical Portions

*Meat – The size of a deck of cards, the palm of your hand, or 3-4 ounces

*Fish – 6-7 ounces

*Vegetables – 1 cup

*Fruit – 1 cup or 1 piece

*Bread – 1 slice, 1 small tortilla, or ½ bagel

*Hot Cereal – ¾ cup cooked

*Cold Cereal – ¾ cup

*Sweet Potato – 1 small baked

*1 Egg

*1 tbsp. Peanut Butter or Cream Cheese

*1 tbsp. Oil

*1/4 Avocado

*5-6 Olives

*1 Cup Clear Soup

*1 Small Bun or Roll

*1 Cup Fresh Squeezed Juice

*5-6 Crackers

*3/4 Cup Pasta, Rice, Quinoa, or Couscous

*1/2 cup hummus

*1/2 cup Low-Fat Frozen Yogurt

*1 Cheese String

*3/4 Cup Yogurt

*1/4 Cup Nuts

*1/4 Cup Raisins

*1/4 Cup Sunflower Seeds

*2-3 tbsp. Seeds (sesame/flax/hemp)

*1-2 tbsp. Low-Fat Dressing

*1/2 Cup Tuna Salad or Egg Salad

*1 Cup Almond Milk

*3/4 Cup Cottage Cheese

*3/4 Cup Sugar-Free Pudding

Chapter 5 - Sugar Down - Energy Up - Appetite Up - Memory Down!

Livestrong.com professionals say sucrose raises energy levels depending on how much you eat. If you have a sugar pig-out session you'll experience a sugar high. This is where your blood glucose levels shoot through the roof with your energy levels, followed by a sharp descent.

Sugar isn't technically a stimulant. However it mimics the common stimulant caffeine.

Psychology Today experts also remind us overeating with sugary foods triggers more overeating, learning disorders, depression, and poor memory overall. Sugar negatively affects your brain.

Energy is Sugar

When your body gets glucose your pancreas injects insulin into your blood stream to eat up the glucose. In this form your brain and body can use it for energy. Any extra glucose is changed into glycogen by the liver and stored in tissues and muscle. As a gauge your body can only hold about 12 hours of glycogen. The rest gets tucked away as fat.

Unless you have a medical condition, hypoglycemia (low blood sugar) is rare. Having high blood sugar triggers heart disease, stroke, nerve damage, and eye issues. It's wise to get your blood sugar levels checked regularly. And for reference a blood sugar reading below 40 mg/deciliter or above 100 mg/deciliter are extremely dangerous.

According to Best Health Magazine specialists high blood sugar levels damage blood vessels, leading to heart health issues. They also tax your memory and trigger specific cancers to develop. The cancer cell thrives on simple sugar carbohydrates. These health issues don't happen immediately but manifest over time. And if you shut excess sugar out of your life you will notice fast energy and more alertness.

Scary Note - Researchers have found that continually dosing your body with large amounts of sugar over a long period of time will damage it even if the consequences don't equate to diabetes.

The silent killer ----

Problem - The sugars we are consuming in insane quantities are added. They don't come from fresh fruits and grains. Instead they are derived from unhealthy processed foods with oodles of fructose. I think of fructose as "the trigger crave."

Up to 10% of your daily caloric intake should be from sugars to help fuel your brain properly. It's the added sugars that kill your energy and body.

People Get Tricked into Eating Sweets for Energy because it's a Quick Reward

When you drink a soda, energy drink, or down a couple candy bars you inject an immediate energy burst that makes you feel good. We like that and want more. Simple refined sugar energy only lasts about 30 minutes before the crash, which isn't a good thing.

If you want long-term sustainable energy you've got to cut out the cupcakes, cookies, cakes pastries, donuts, vending machine sandwiches, and other processed boxed and packaged foods and replace them with healthy natural sugars. These are found in a balanced diet of fresh fruits and veggies, healthy whole grain bread, pasta and rice, and good fats found in coconut oil and olive oil.

VEGAN ALERT!!!

The Vegan Diet is an excellent route for cutting out added sugars and building your body and mind strong, and paying respect to the environment and all the creatures of the earth. Energy levels soar with vegan eating because processed sugary foods are removed and you are always eating healthy nutrient loaded fibrous foods.

Even when practicing a wholesome vegan lifestyle you need to be aware of what you are eating and make sure sugar hasn't been added.

Tips to Increase Energy Vegan Style by Cutting Sugar

Focus Fat - You'll curb your sugar cravings by boosting healthy fats.

Choose to eat:

*Avocado - In salads and stir-fry, smoothies, soups, and dressings.

*Nuts - Sprinkle on cereal, in salads, yogurts and stew, and eat with dried fruit.

*Mixed Seeds - Flax, hemp, chia, and sesame seeds are tasty in anything from salads and veggies, to sauces and cereals.

*Olive Oil and Coconut Oil are great on salads or drizzled on cooked veggies and meats.

Plenty of Healthy Protein - Since you've cut out complete animal fat protein out of your diet it's important you eat plenty of different protein sources to get all 20 amino acids each day. Proteins help keep your hormones in line and sugar cravings asleep.

Choose to eat:

*Plenty of Legumes and Beans

*Nuts and Seeds

*Spirulina - A great source of protein that's great in a smoothie.

*Grains - Quinoa is excellent because it's the only plant based protein that's complete.

Your aim is to eat all-natural REAL foods as close to Mother Nature as possible. This removes all extra sugars, prevents disease, and boosts your energy levels. But this means you've got to commit to taking all your fast-food eating out of the equation. This includes sprinkling sugar on your berries and cereal, loading your morning coffee with sweet stuff, and choosing a natural tea in the afternoon instead of your usual sugar packed flavored fancy beverage.

Change is good and getting rid of sugar is especially good to change your energy levels and drive them upward to stay. Not just for short unstable bursts.

Chapter 6 - Key Benefits of Kicking Sugar Out

I'm sure you don't need any convincing that unnatural ADDED sugars are bad news. They make you fat and increase your risk of serious disease like cancer, diabetes, heart disease and stroke.

*There is no silver lining with refined sugar.

Sugar-Free Eating Will Benefit You Mentally and Physically By:

Decreasing Your Risk of Sickness and Disease

Added sugar steals nutrients required for optimal metabolic function. This triggers nutrient deficient disease like osteoporosis, iron deficiencies, and immune issues. Sugar also triggers growth of hormones with insulin release. Your blood cells are forced to clean up the waste left behind by sugar instead of protect your body from invading free radicals.

Add this this sugar weakens your intestinal tract so nutrients aren't readily absorbed and dispersed properly. Bloating and gas are notable symptoms.

Empowering You to Take Control of Cravings and Hunger

Nutrient stores are depleted when sugar is on the menu. Some of which are used to help control inflammation. Sugar doesn't contain essential macronutrients and micronutrients necessary for good health. Good fat, lean protein, and healthy complex carbs are required to satiate your hunger and nip cravings in the bud. Sugar interferes with this and leaves your body and mind unsatisfied and confused.

Sugar is addictive and you can never get enough. One donut leads to three or four because you are not communicating to your brain that your hunger is satisfied because you pumping yourself full of foreign substances your brain and body don't know how to interpret or use. It's a cyclical process where your blood sugars get bounced around and the easy answer is to keep eating more sugar to temporarily feel good. Then when you get dumped to the bottom of the barrel you crave more sweet stuff to climb out.

Eliminating sugars balances blood sugars, reducing cravings and controlling hunger!

Boosting Energy

WebMD medical expert's state sugar slows you down. When you eat it your energy levels spike. Blood sugars shoot up and insulin is released. When insulin is released so is tryptophan which converts to serotonin, and sets you up for a nice nap.

By eating a healthy diet loaded with protective antioxidants from fresh fruits and berries, vitamins, minerals, fiber, water, complex carbs, and protein to fuel your mind, you fly through your day instead of ridding your tiresome sugar roller coaster of constant ups and downs.

Sharpen Thinking

Scientists have no doubt sugar negatively affects your thought process. Excess refined sugar interferes with memory and fools with concentration. It also triggers negative thinking and unnatural nervousness. When you consume sugar even in small doses you are altering your brain chemistry. And there's no room for that in healthy living.

Find You, Set Healthy Weight and Stay There

You were born with in internal set weight where your body functioned optimally. Unfortunately life got in the way and you likely stressed your body so much your weight reset much higher than is truly healthy for you. By removing the interference of sugar you will naturally encourage your body to shed fat, assuming you are eating healthy and exercising, so you can find your healthy weight range and stay there.

It's a safe bet that knocking extra sugar out of your diet is going to trigger weight loss fast!

Look Better

Sugar steals nutrients you need to look and feel fantastic. Sugar experts report when sugar attaches to protein it's called glyceration. This takes the blame for wrinkles, saggy skin, and a dull complexion.

Deter Allergies

It's no big secret many allergies are triggered by foreign substances or processed sugary foods. Experts believe people with sensitive systems that subject themselves to extra sugars and processed food additives increase their risk of developing food sensitivities or food allergies.

Less Cavities

I'm sure your dentist has told you point blank that sugar rots teeth. Sugar actually invites bacteria growth that develops into cavities. Stay away from sugar for better dental hygiene.

Positive Thinking

When you are on the sugary moody roller coaster it's difficult to stay level and focus on the positive. By eliminating sugar you give your body a chance to find balance in thinking and function. Your constant energized mood will light up your world instead of flood it with dark clouds. The "thehealthyhomeeconomist.com" suggest by 2020 major depression will become a disability with up to 25% of the population suffering from it. Sugar is a direct cause because it destabilizes the brain through glycation. Knock out the sugars and you've a fighting chance to smile permanently.

Getting Rid of Headaches, Aches and Pains

Experts agree sugar causes inflammation and this creates aches, pains, and disease. By reducing or removing sugar from your diet you'll feel a weight lifted off your shoulders, literally.

SAMPLE SUGAR-FREE MEALS

Breakfast

*2 eggs poached, 1 slice whole grain toast, 1 glass fresh squeezed juice

*1 cup cooked oatmeal with 1 cup fresh berries, 1 cup fruit, coffee

*1 tbsp. all-natural peanut butter in whole grain wrap with sliced banana, 1 cup chunked grapefruit, tea

*I cup all-natural yogurt with 1/4 cup sliced almond and 1/4 cup sunflower seeds, banana, orange, coffee

Lunch

*Grilled chicken wrapped in whole wheat tortilla with shredded cheese, cucumber, tomato, spinach, sprouts, and water chestnuts, apple, lemon water

*3/4 cup whole grain pasta with 1/4 cup no sugar tomato sauce, 1 small whole grain bun, 1 cup steamed veggies

*3/4 cup cottage cheese with 1/2 cup pineapple, cheese string and banana

*Half a rye pita stuffed with tuna salad, cucumber, lettuce, tomato, green pepper, and sprouts, 2 cups spinach salad with drizzle olive oil

Dinner

*Grilled salmon with steamed asparagus, baked sweet potato

*2 cups grilled peppers, carrots, zucchini, broccoli, asparagus, bok choy, 3/4 cup lentils, 1 cup fresh fruit

*Small portion barbecued steak, 3/4 cup legumes, 2 cups spinach salad with 1/4 cup oranges and 1/4 cup sliced almonds

*2 cups Romaine lettuce topped with 1 cup steamed quinoa, 1 cup steamed broccoli, 1/4 cup sunflower seeds, 1/4 cup sliced almonds, banana

NOTE: Be careful with your cooking. Make sure you check the labels on everything and don't use bottled sauces. Lemons and olive oil or coconut oil work great for cooking and adding flavor. You can teach your taste buds to crave "naked." That's a great thing.

These meal ideas show you just how easy it is to eat minus the sugar. It takes awareness and preparation but where there's a will there's a way. And on the flip side of all these benefits there's really nothing advantageous about adding sugar into your diet. There are only immediate consequences and ones further down the road while you play your game of Russian roulette by including loads of sugar into your diet. Your health is your most prized possession. You owe it to yourself to do whatever it takes to kick sugar out of your life for good and bask in the glory of amazing long-term health and wellness.

Conclusion

Livescience experts report in 2013 sugary drinks were linked to over 180,000 deaths worldwide. That's just the tip of the iceberg. Fructose is the most deadly because of its scientifically proven addictive powers. And the fact it makes up half of the sugars in processed foods.

The sugars found in cakes, muffins, donuts, pastries, cookies, white bread products, and pretty much any bagged, boxed, or packaged food, are deadly in time. They will interfere with weight loss, your mood and physical appearance, they'll make you fat, interfere with clear thinking, steal energy, and increase your risk of developing serious disease like diabetes, cancer, heart disease, stroke, and Alzheimer's.

By gathering the take-action information you need to eliminate harmful added sugar from your diet you will literally receive a new lease on life. Leveling your blood sugars sooner not later is a smooth move.

When you are ready to commit to sugar-free living you now have the information to get you started. Good Luck!

See bonus chapter on next page

BONUS CHAPTER - Physiological Behind Sugar Addiction

Kelly McGonigal, health psychologist Stanford reminds us that both the mind and body are addicted to sugar. Usually an addictive substance starts by releasing a substance that makes you feel good. And when you feel this pleasure, energy, or warm focus you naturally want more.

Truth is your body and brain are looking to keep your internal systems running smooth because of homeostasis, where your physical and thinking mechanisms adapt.

A good example is where you eat a bag of candy and your serotonin levels shoot up. Your brain's defense mechanism is to reduce the number of receptors for this substance so it has less effect and more balance. This is your body naturally fighting the heightened effects of this particular substance. And what this does is make you want more to get a more satisfying effect.

With time this process gains momentum and you begin experiencing stronger cravings and use more of the substance, in this case sugar, to get the experienced desired effect.

Study One

Psychology Today reports a study done with mice to show this effect. Mice were given a sweet that triggered their brain to release orexin. In mice this substance causes the muscles to absorb the sweet for the expected blood sugar rise. This is natural adaptation.

So when they tried to resist temptations the blood sugar levels dropped which increased the physical want for the sweet, the craving. You see this in babies when you give them blended apricots instead of bland beans.

Study Two

Another study was done where students were given a box of chocolates easily visible on their desk, slightly concealed inside the desk, and tucked away a short distance away.

The students with the chocolates on their desk where they could see ate more than the others. Suggesting your vision triggers emotions that makes you want the sweets. So by taking better control of the foods around you its possible to curb sugar cravings and decrease consumption.

Out of sight, out of mind seems to work!

If we see we naturally want. It puts the thought in our head to start craving. Your brain takes the thought and turns it into a physical desire and craving. The craving is what you act on.

This reiterates how important it is to remove all signs of the sugar stimulus when you are vamoosing sugar from your diet. It doesn't help anyway having candy bars on the table or hidden under your bed. Same as it doesn't help to hold an empty water bottle when you are parched and there isn't any water nearby. That just triggers your desire to increase and become more of a focus.

Take Action Steps

*Remove sugar from your environment

*Remove sugar from your daily eating

*Remove sugar from your body with a sugar detox cleanse

Sustain this for 1 month and you've just proven to yourself you can beat sugar!

Do you want to be super healthy for life? Then feel free to read a copy of my "Vegan diet for Beginners" book. Busting sugar cravings has great benefits that come along with it. Wouldn't it be 10 times greater if you switched to a plant based diet? Yes, I know - going vegan is not the easiest decision to make especially if you love eating meat and processed food – I've been there too! However, I have taken time out to make it a lot easier for you. So don't stop there! Don't give up now! You can do this! I believe in you!

 Grab your copy NOW!

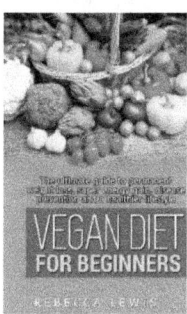

www.ingramcontent.com/pod-product-compliance
Lightning Source LLC
Chambersburg PA
CBHW070843290526
45795CB00002B/960